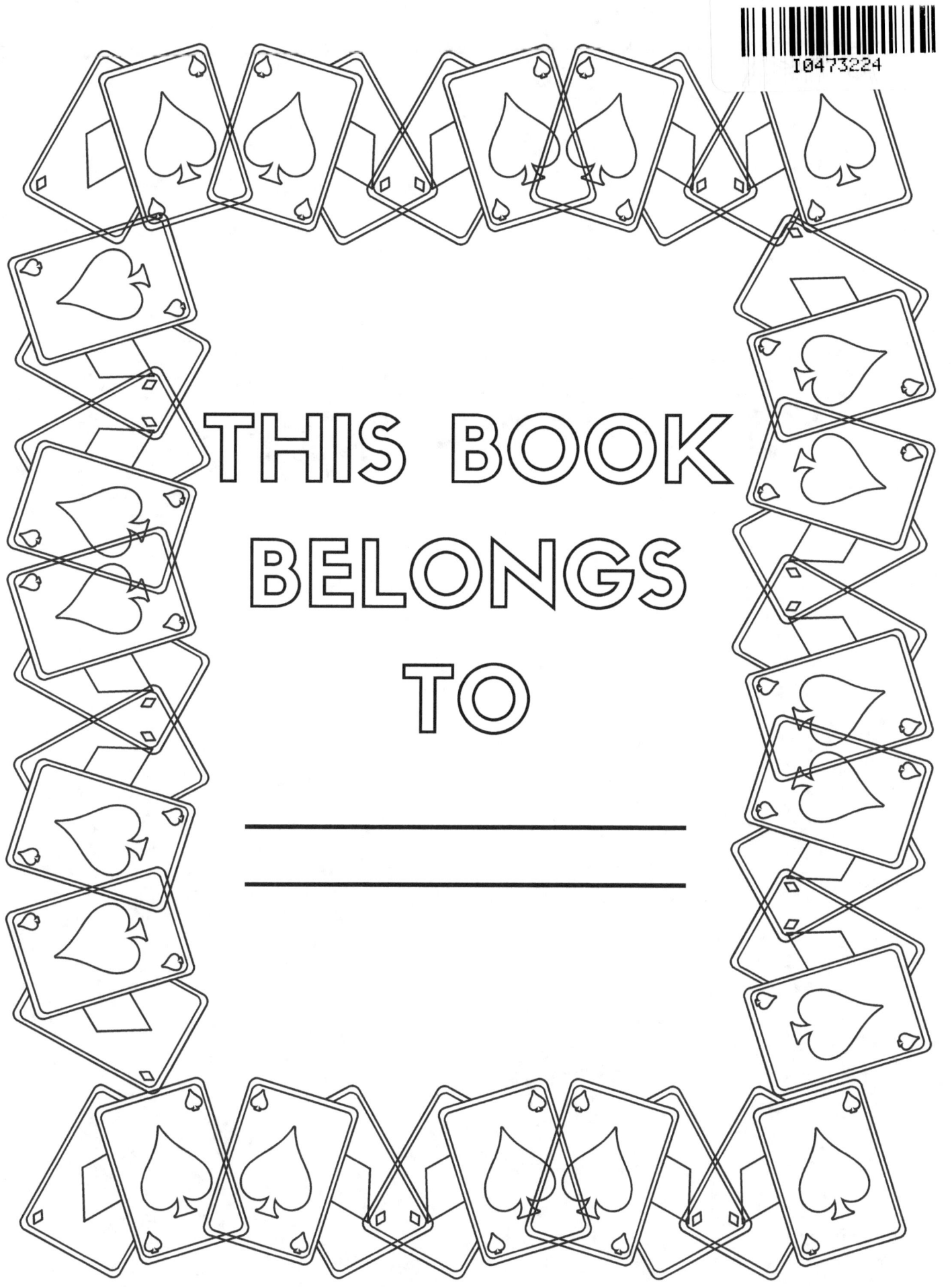

THIS BOOK BELONGS TO

_____
_____

I0473224

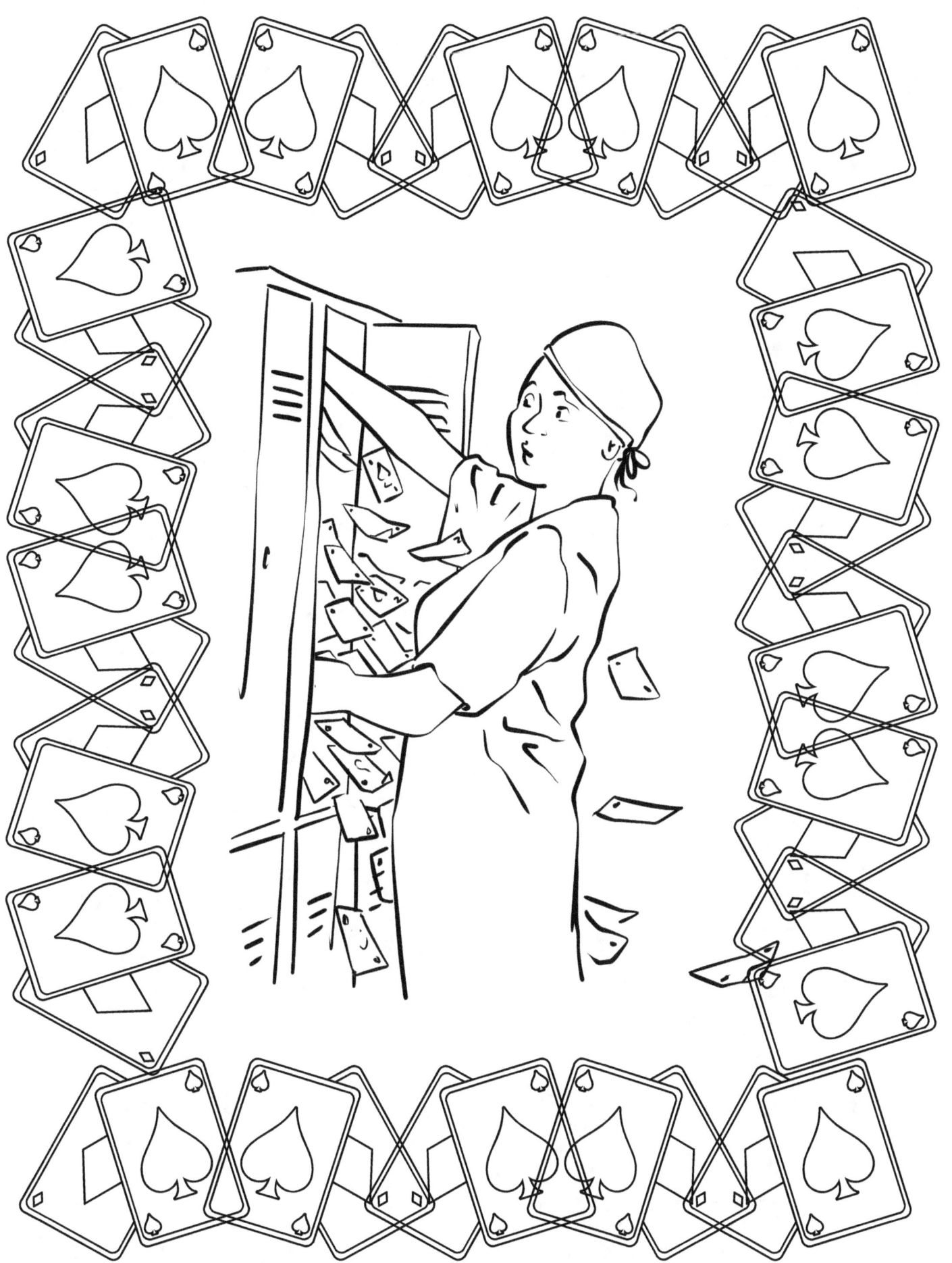

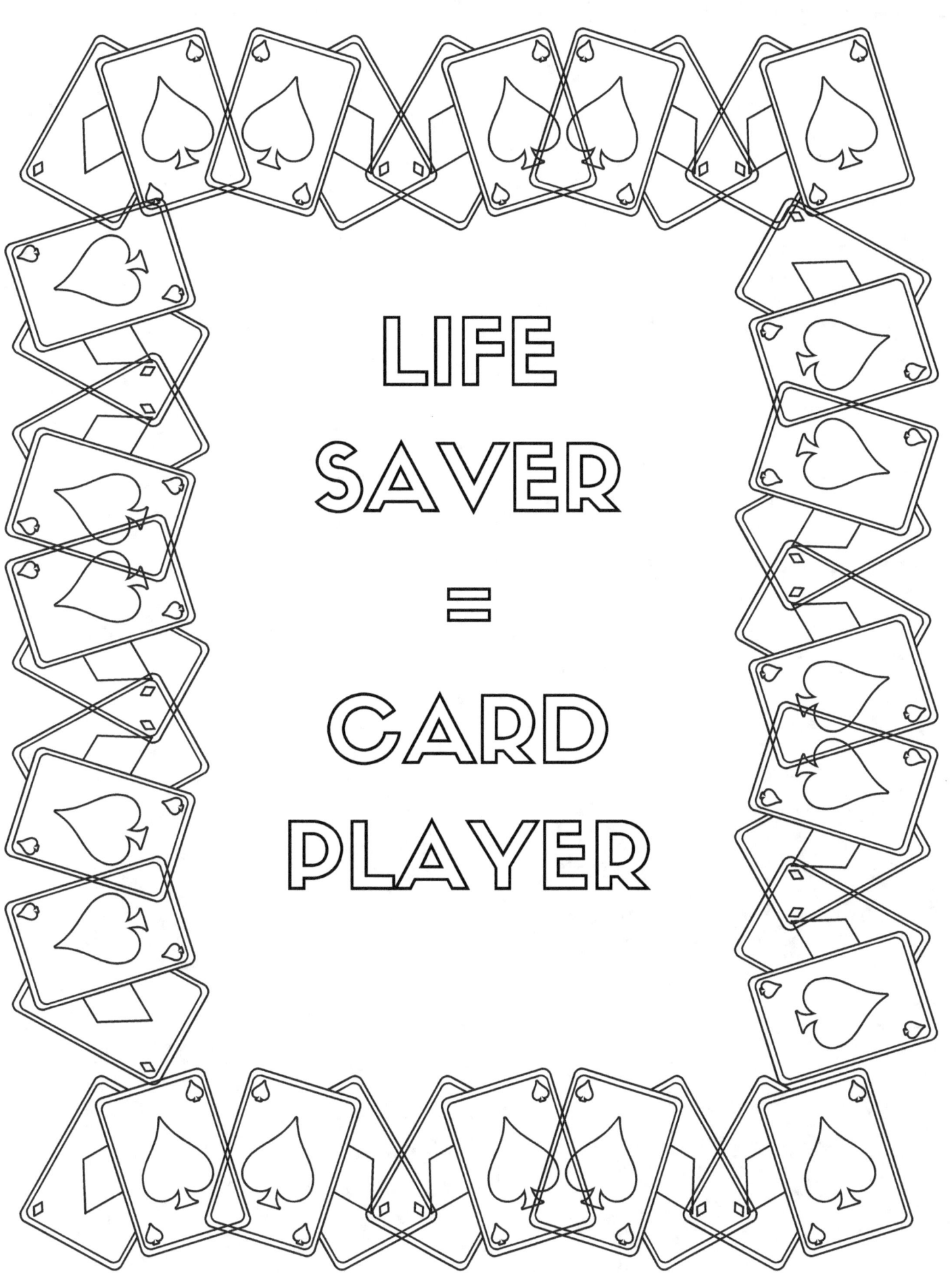

LIFE
SAVER

=

CARD
PLAYER

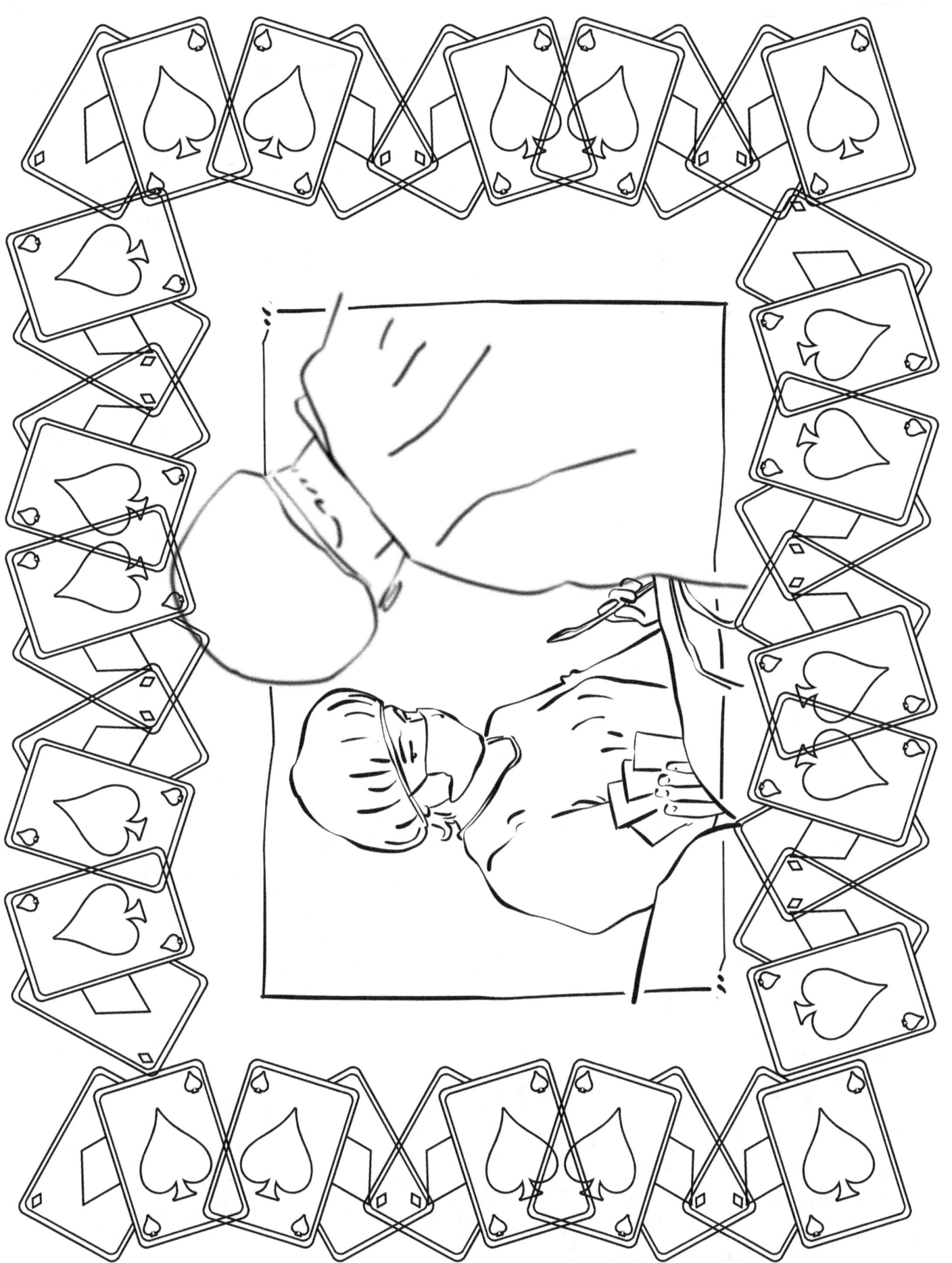

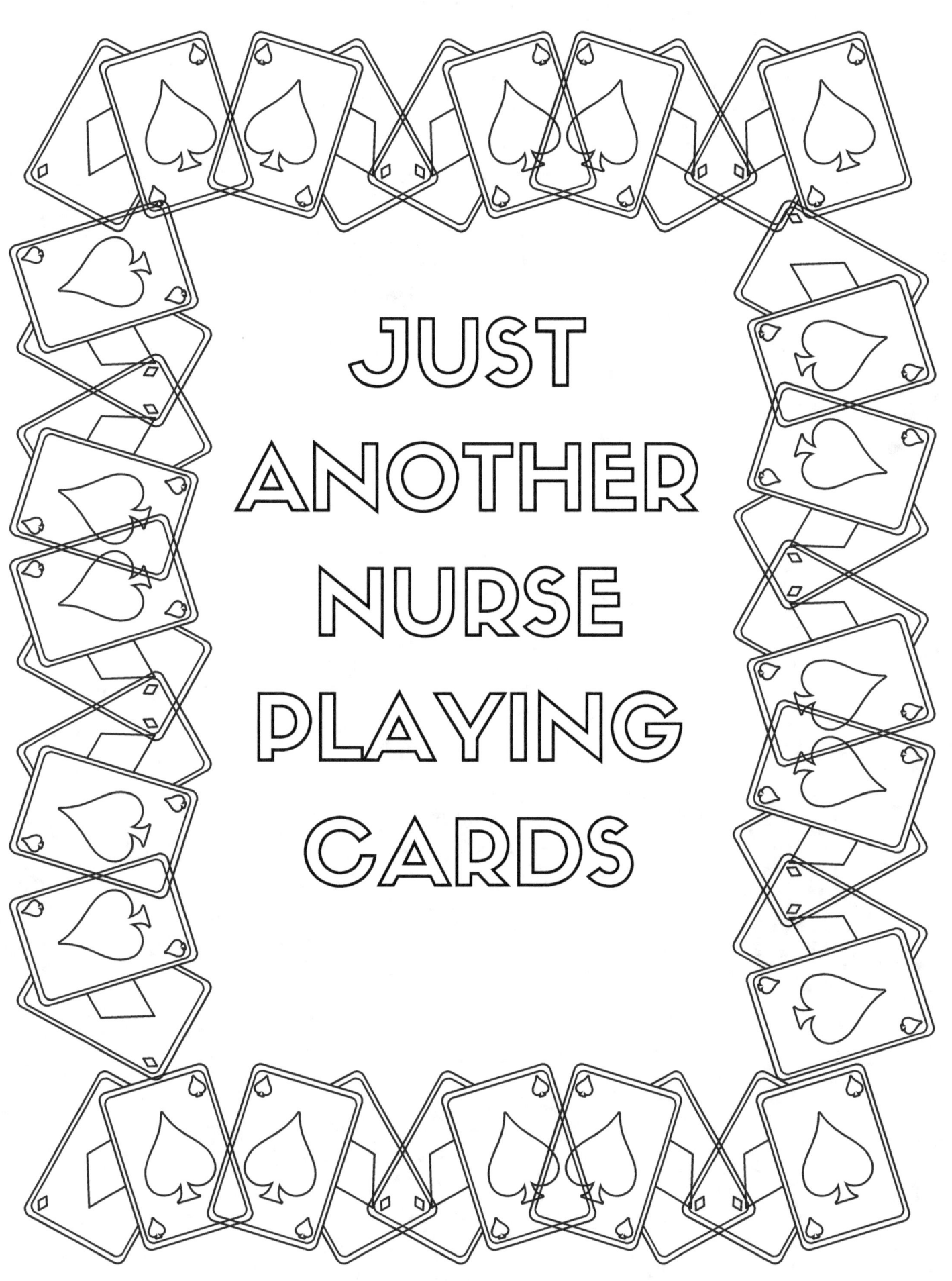

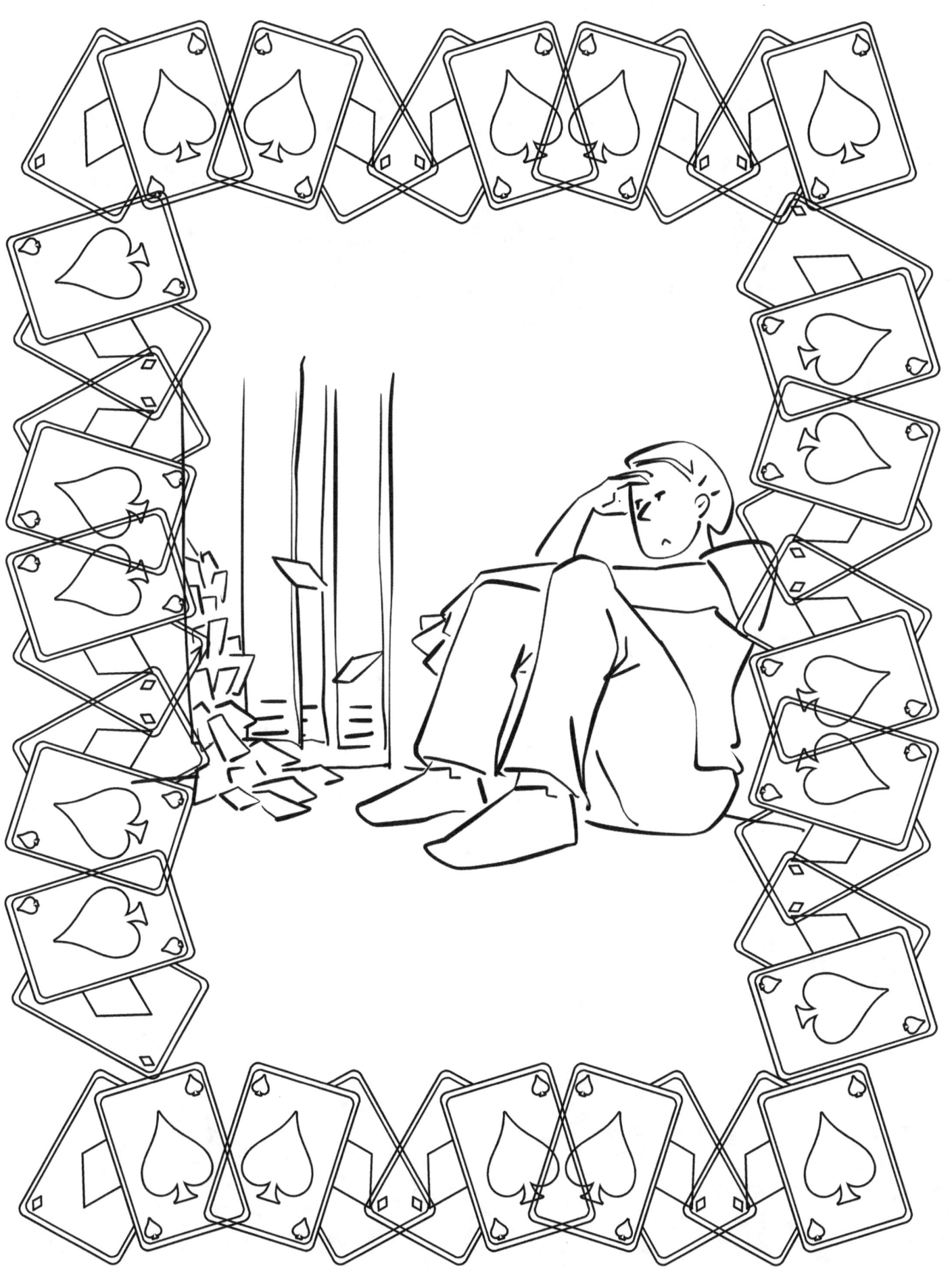

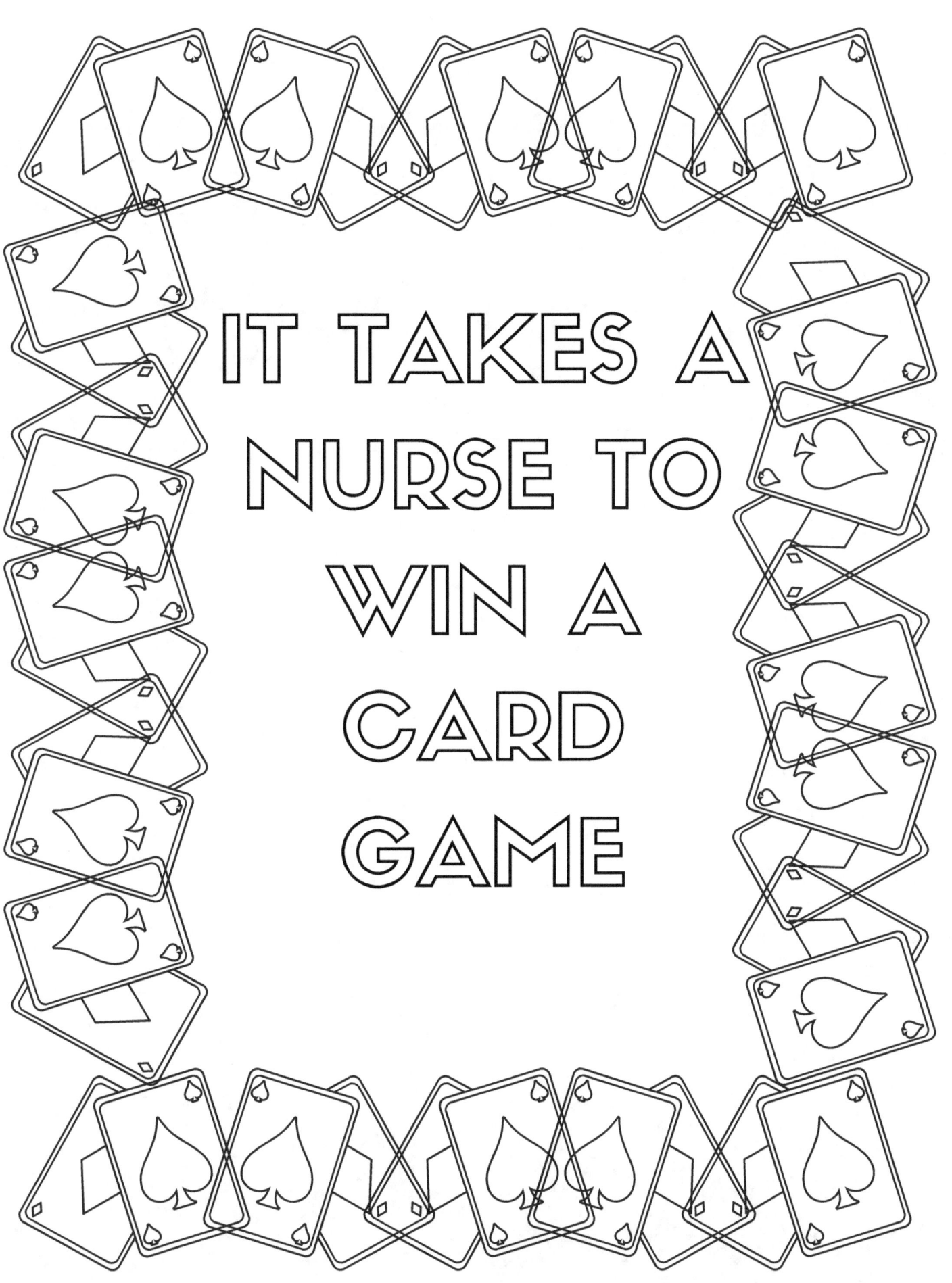

IT TAKES A NURSE TO WIN A CARD GAME

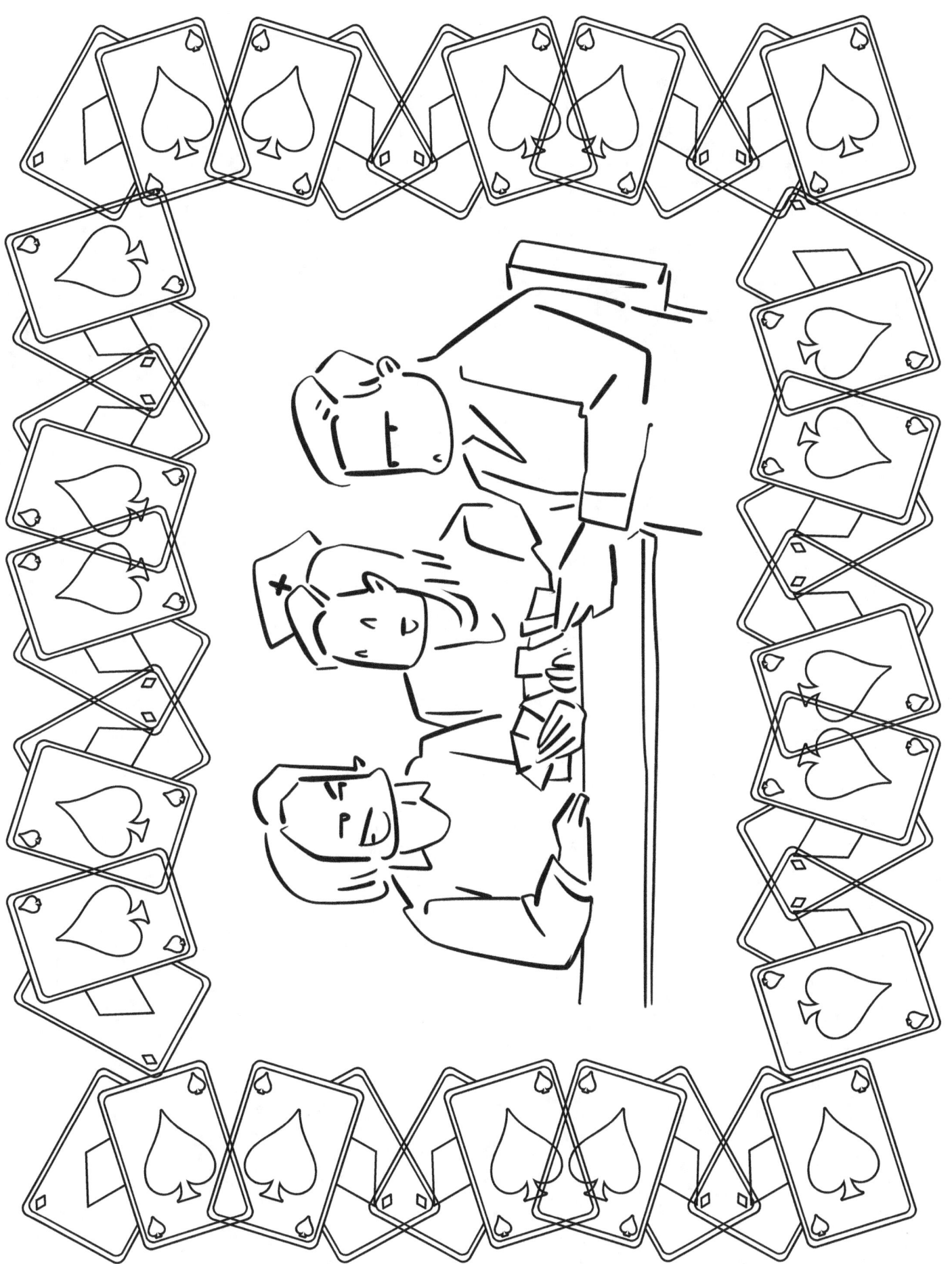

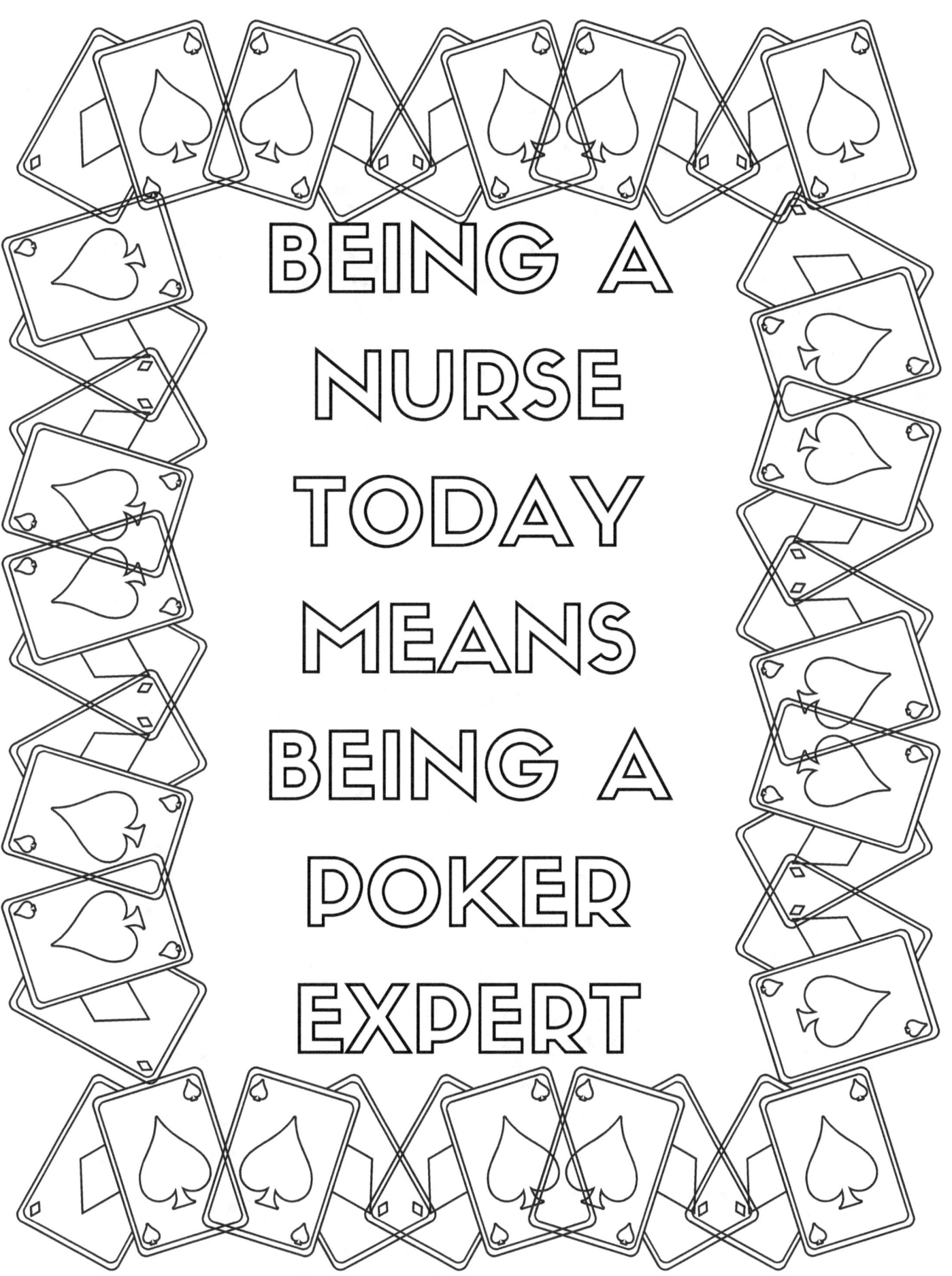

BEING A NURSE TODAY MEANS BEING A POKER EXPERT

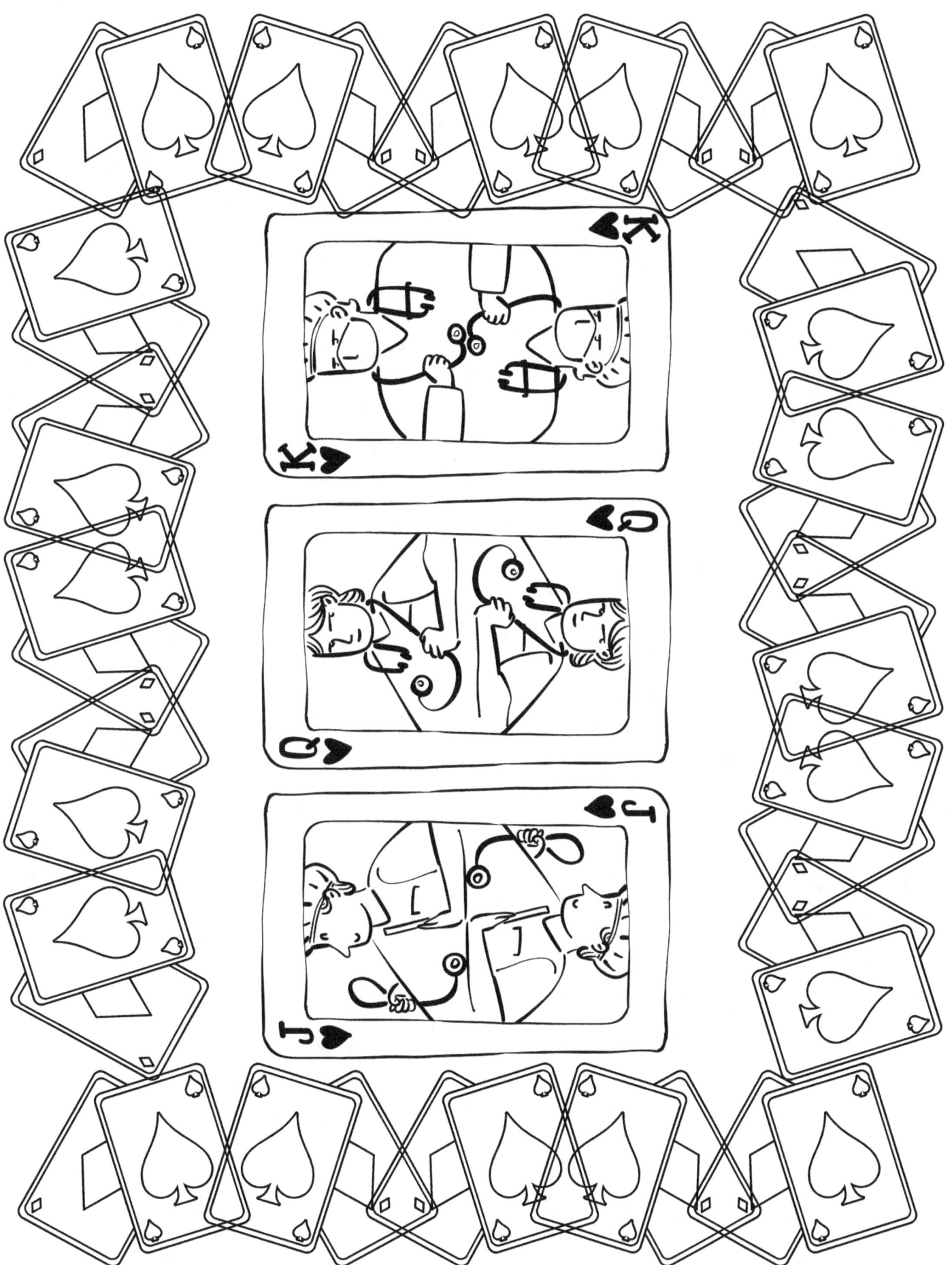

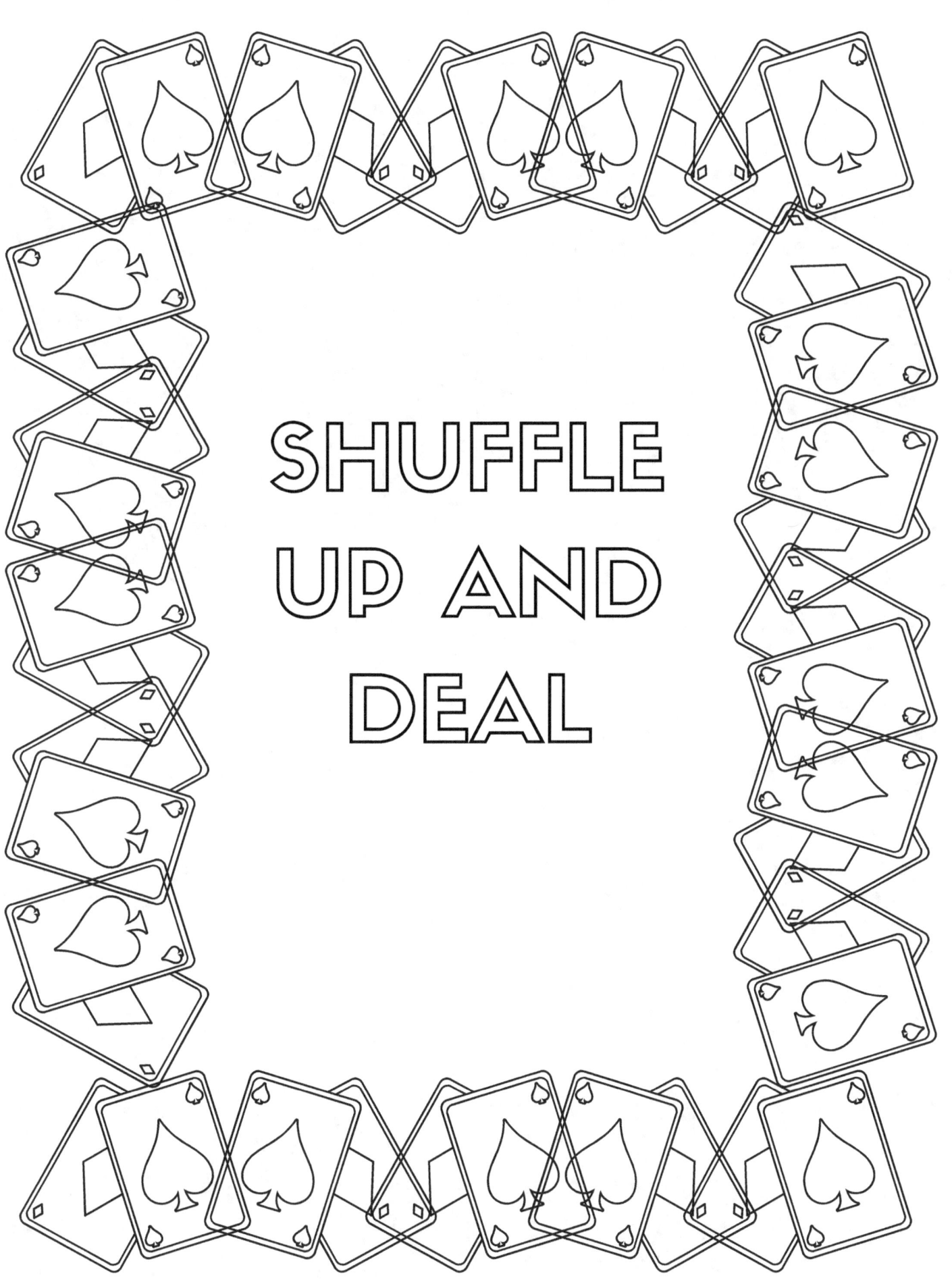

SHUFFLE
UP AND
DEAL

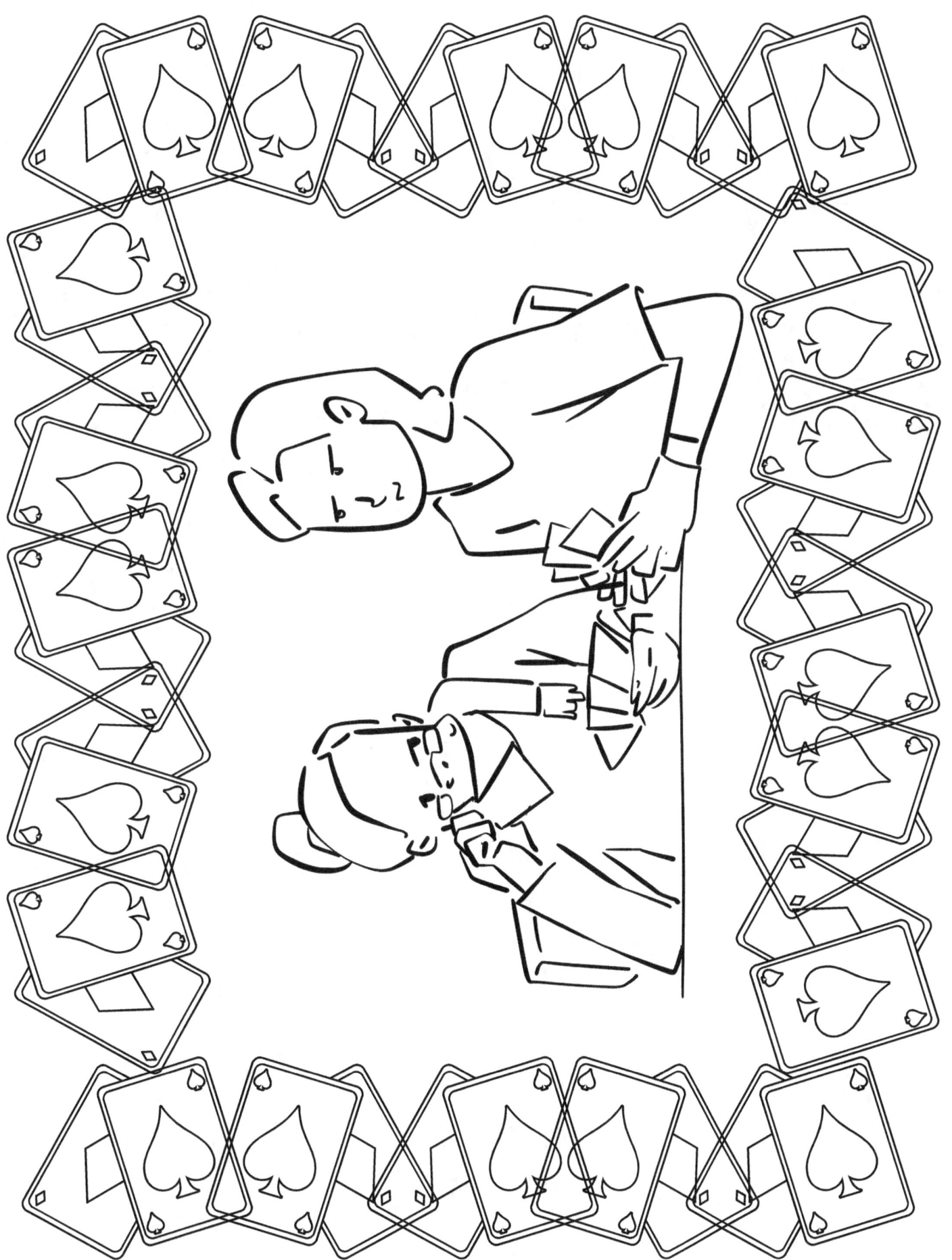

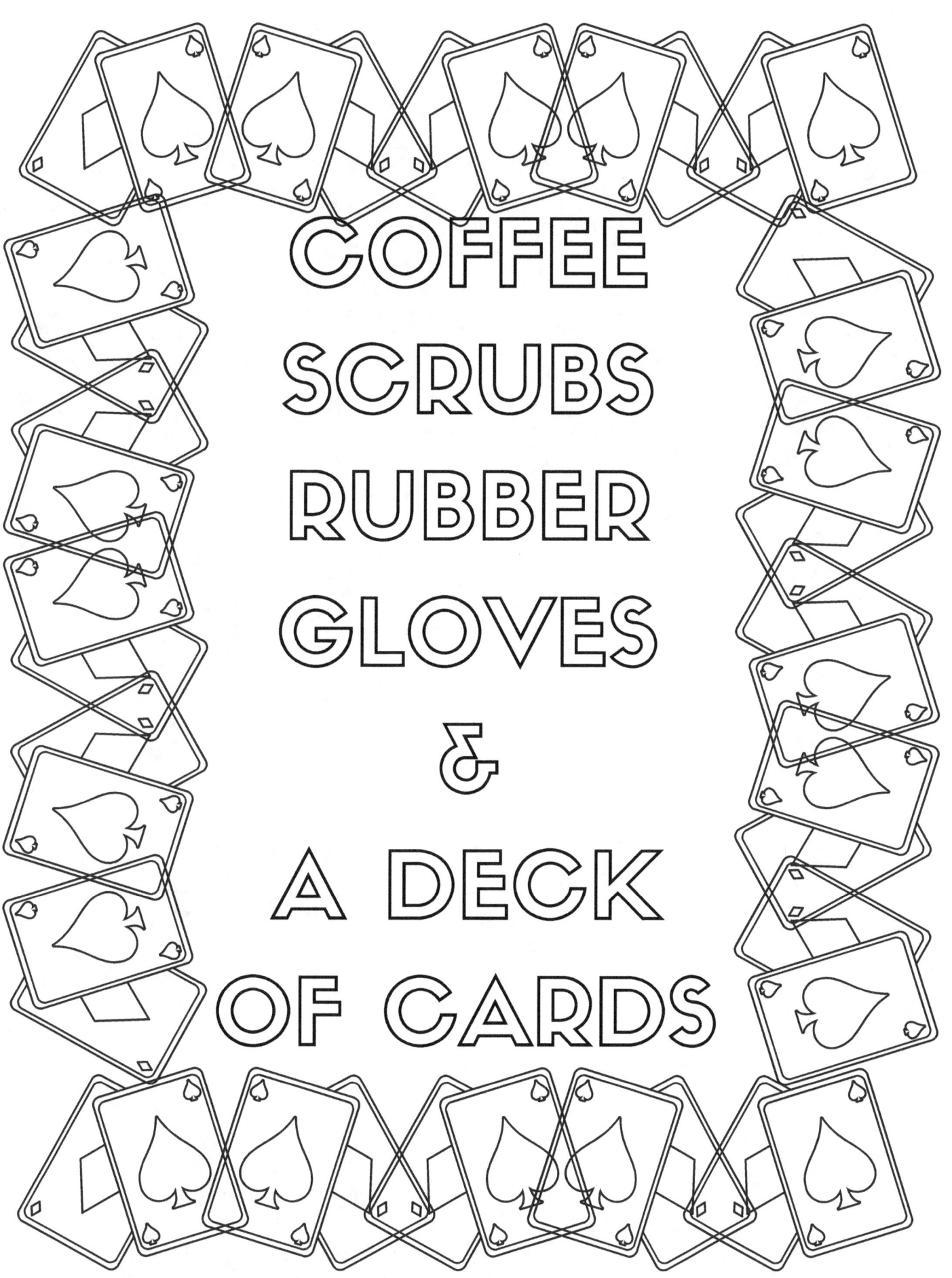

COFFEE
SCRUBS
RUBBER
GLOVES
&
A DECK
OF CARDS

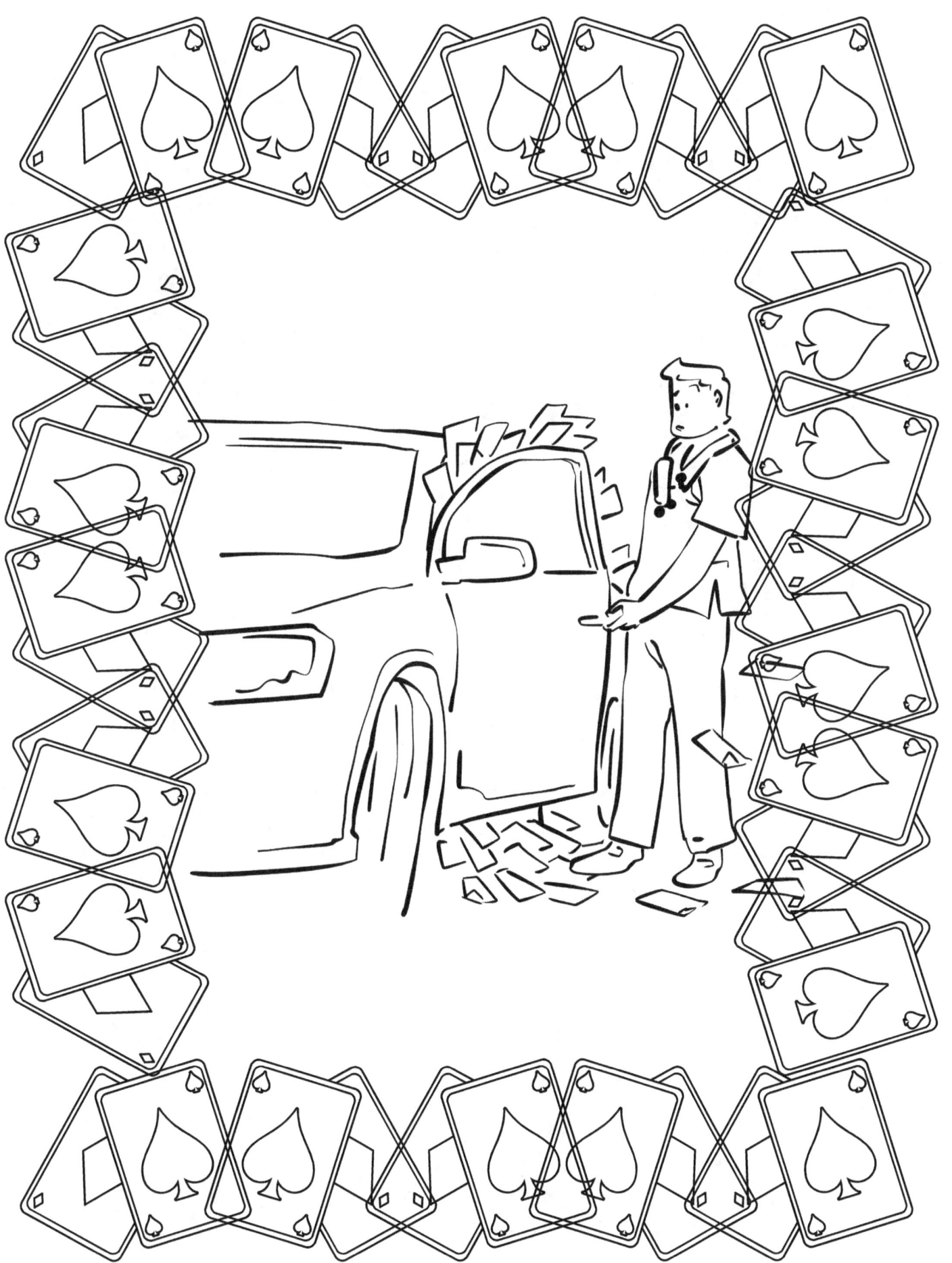

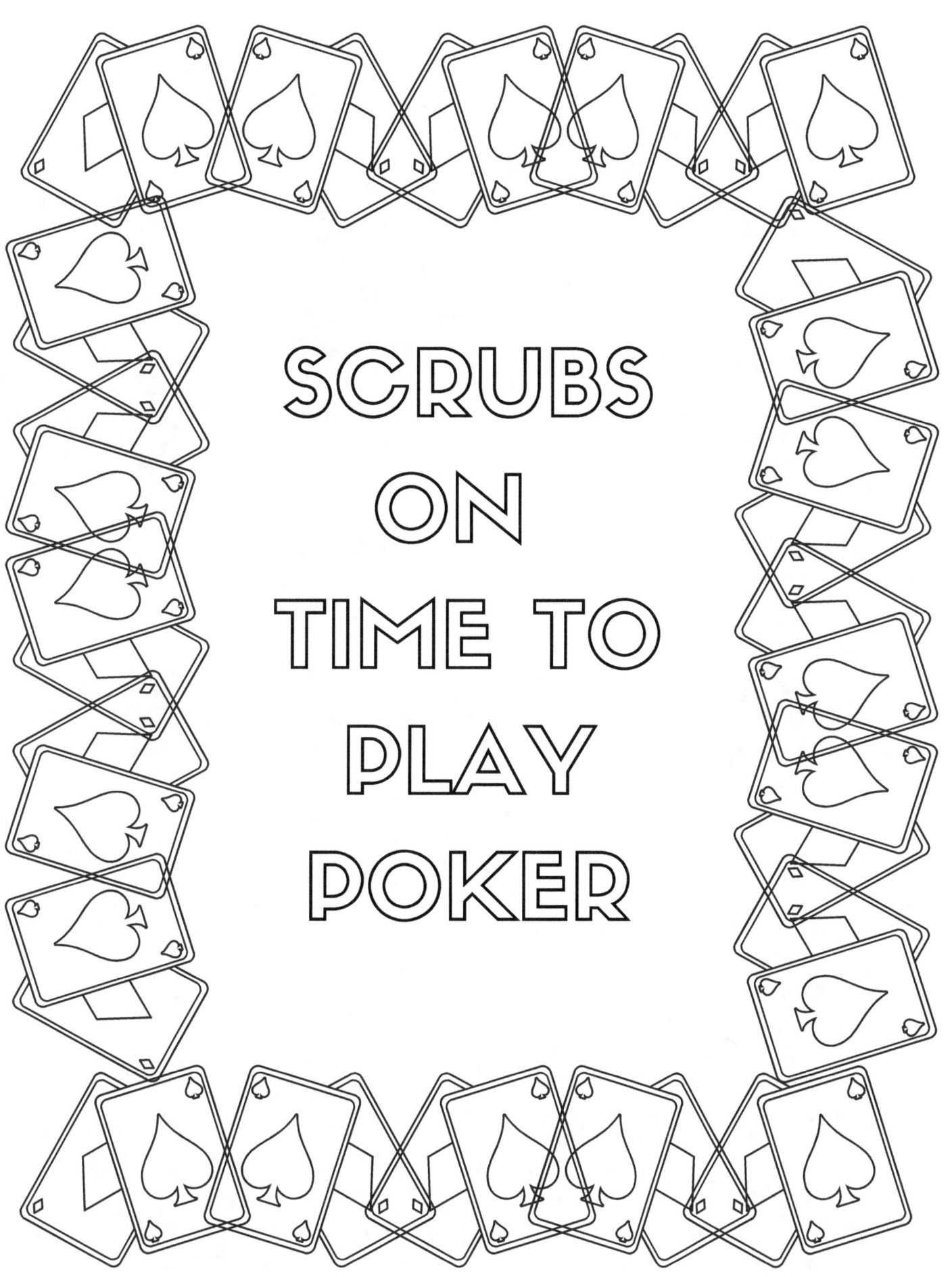

SCRUBS
ON
TIME TO
PLAY
POKER

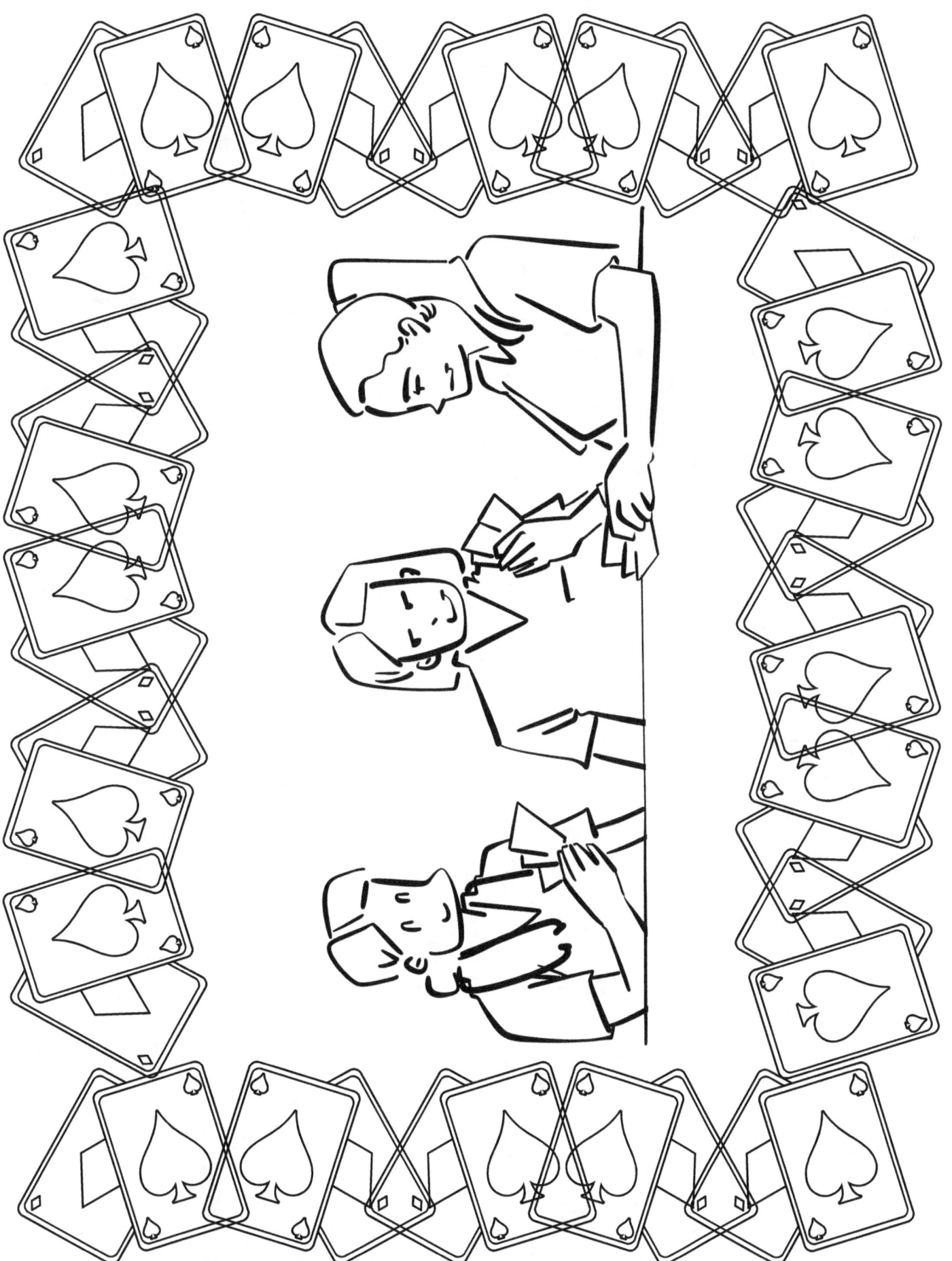

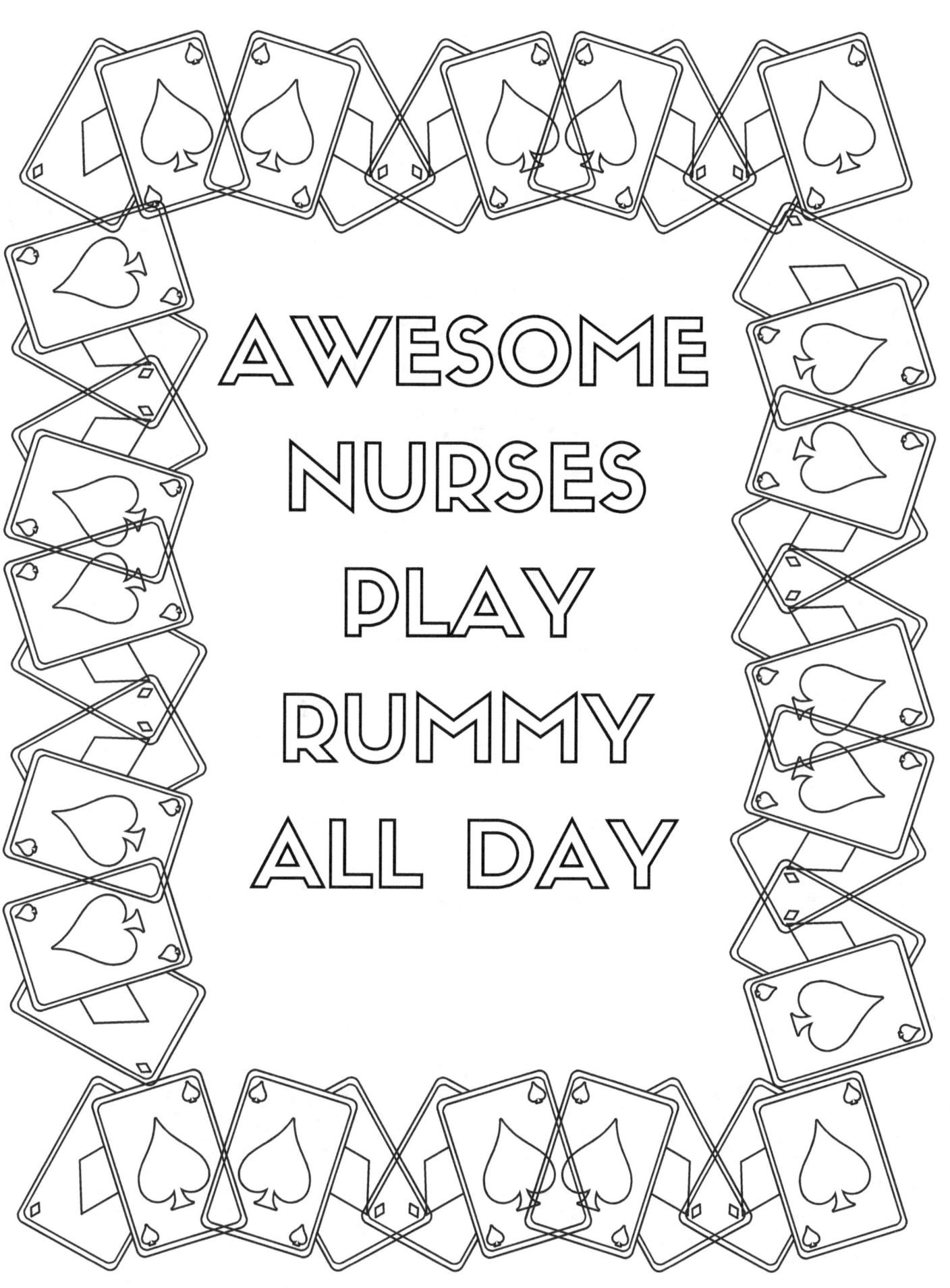

AWESOME NURSES PLAY RUMMY ALL DAY

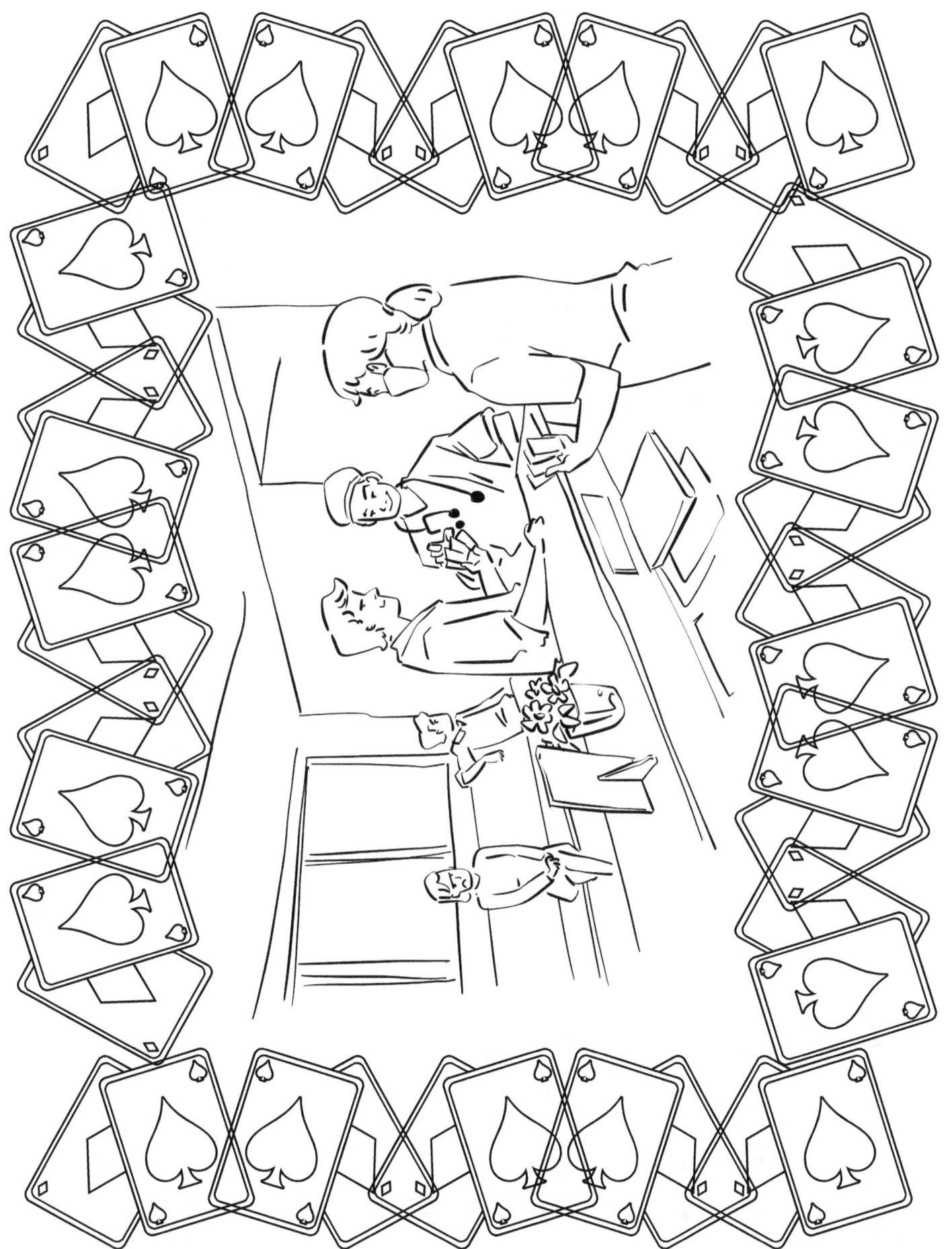

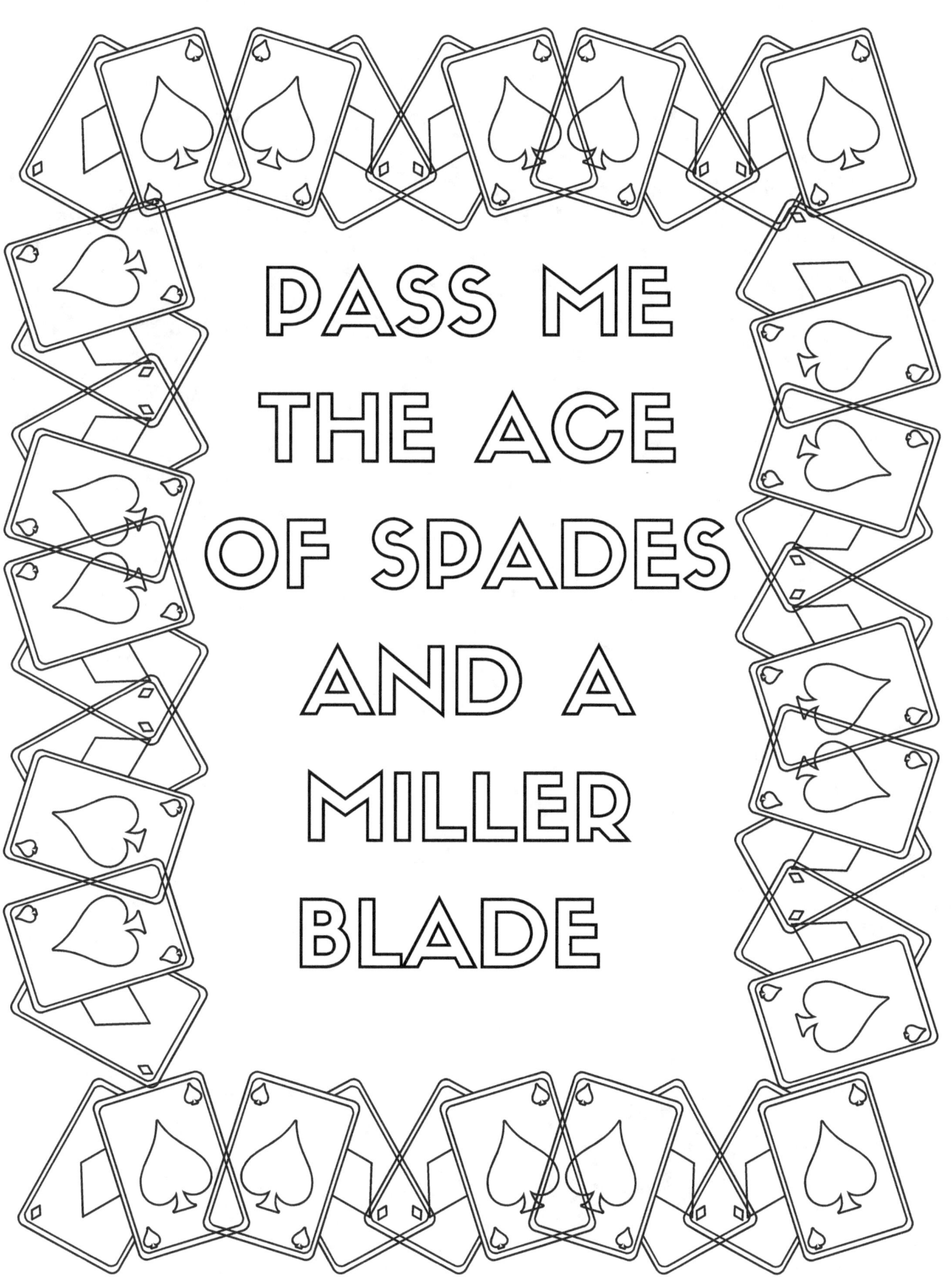

PASS ME
THE ACE
OF SPADES
AND A
MILLER
BLADE

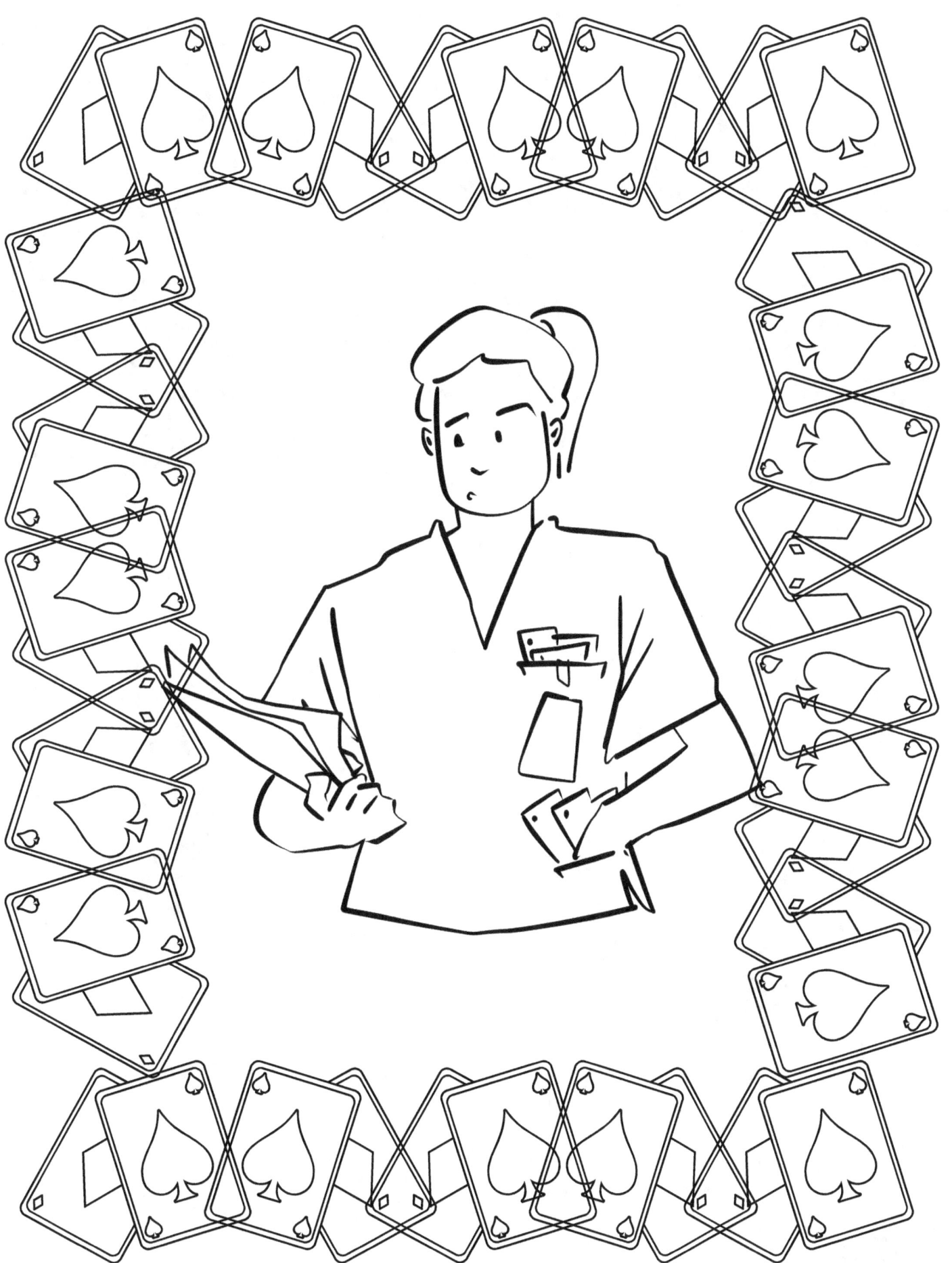

www.ingramcontent.com/pod-product-compliance
Lightning Source LLC
Chambersburg PA
CBHW081147170526
45158CB00009BA/2734